I0407158

It's Not Your Time

By Paul Gagliardi
And Kevin Gerou

PAUL GAGLIARDI

ISBN:1470010224
ISBN-13: 978-1470010225

DEDICATION

I dedicate *It's Not Your Time* to all those who helped me during my struggle with cancer. I owe my life to great doctors, my family, friends, my special friend Nina and all of you who prayed so hard for my recovery. I will never be able to repay you. Thank you for giving me the strength to continue my life. I hope it continues to be worthy of all your efforts.

I want to thank my son Frank Gagliardi for working so hard to keep our law practice going as this was a tremendous stress for him; my son Paul M. Gagliardi in keeping me focused on the message of helping others get through life with cancer; and my daughter Gennie Gerou for helping with the cover and offering great ideas to better convey my message. Thank God she got her design and art talents from her Nana and her mother! I also want to thank all who helped me through the re-writes especially Charlotte Calhoun.

I especially want to thank my son-in-law, Kevin Gerou. Kevin's father Tim was my lifelong friend. Tim lost his battle with cancer shortly before I was diagnosed. I can't imagine how hard it was for him to assist in this endeavor. Without Kevin's skill and ability, my rambling thoughts would not have left the computer. Kevin is a talented writer and musician as well as being a great son-in-law.

Also want to thank my special friend, Nancy Swenson for her patience and assistance helping complete this project.

PAUL GAGLIARDI

PAUL GAGLIARDI

CONTENTS

FORWARD

Everyone is motivated in different ways. Ron Bachman is a famous motivational speaker whose birth defect cost him his legs at the age of four. He could have felt sorry for himself and given up on his goals – but he didn't. Everyone diagnosed with cancer has the same choice to either fight for a healthy life or simply give up. Every person who has a loved one diagnosed with cancer can say, "Why me?" Whether to fight for a healthy life or not is your choice.

There are no rules of fairness in life. You get what is dished out and play the cards you are dealt. Each person plays cards his or her own way. *It's Not Your Time* is the story of how I played my hand when my doctors told my son to have his father get his stuff in order and added, "Your father has a deadly cancer and only has 30 to 60 days to live."

I didn't believe I was dying. All my life, I only knew how to play to win. I told my family to give me a chance to fight this cancer. I told the doctors they had my chart mixed up with someone else's. I wasn't really sick. Maybe I just got a spider bite!

However, deep down I knew what I was facing. I knew this life could be over soon and it wasn't my call. It wasn't for me to decide and I didn't have control. The deck had shuffled. There was one thing that I knew though: folding wasn't an option.

The goal behind *It's Not Your Time* is to provide some insight on how to block out the obstacles that keep you from focusing all your strength and energy on getting well. This is how I found enough strength to fight cancer.

Nick Cetta, a doctor and friend, suggested that I write about how I approached my diagnosis. Since Nick believes positive thinking is the best medicine in the world, he wanted me to share my experience with others facing a potentially fatal illness themselves. He feels my story will benefit others. I also wanted to share my good fortune; hopefully, what helped me will help you.

WHY ME?

I've had a lot of friends and clients that have asked the "Why me?" question after being diagnosed with cancer. I am a trial lawyer who has handled many delayed diagnosis cancer cases. In a delayed diagnosis case, if the doctor doesn't diagnose the cancer in a timely manner within the medical standard of care, he is considered negligent. The problem with these cases is what we lawyers call "the causation question." Has the delay made a difference? If the patient is destined to die regardless of when being diagnosed, there is no case. It is like someone taking a swing at you but missing. We commonly refer to this as "no harm - no foul."

I know the odds for cancer patients surviving. I had to in order to evaluate my cases. We can't accurately predict who will get cancer and who won't but overall, an alarming number of us are afflicted with cancer. Our bodies are complex. Our cells reproduce at rates that the human mind really can't comprehend. Since cancer is the condition where the bad cells kill the good cells, we can call it a numbers game. The bad cells reproduce faster than the good cells until they out number them. In effect, the bad cells suffocate the good cells.

Normally, our body functions the opposite way. The good cells destroy the bad cells. However, no process is perfect and this includes the natural reproduction of the cells that make up human tissue. Bad cells are created all the time. It is only when the bad cells outnumber the good cells that they take over and we can lose the battle.

This battle is growing into a deadly war against mankind. The yearly cancer-related deaths exceeded 1.5 million in 2011 for just the United States alone. The medical costs could feed a third world country. The pain and despair from the loss of loved ones is not even measurable. I suspect you understand this pain if you are reading this book.

The next time you go to church or to a movie, look to your left and then to your right. One or more of the three of you will have cancer at some point in your life. You may have cancer whether you know it or not. Unfortunately, this is how common cancer is.

Some cancers are more deadly than others and we know there are changes we can make to help us against the odds. Unfortunately, no matter what we do, no one can run or hide from cancer. I followed the rules. I didn't smoke. I exercised regularly. I watched what I ate. Yet, I still was afflicted by cancer.

One day, I began to feel tired and I didn't have time to be fatigued. For one thing, I had an important trip to Washington, D.C. I was scheduled to meet with members of Congress regarding important issues that affected people back home in

Wisconsin. I was the president-elect for the Wisconsin Association for Justice and I had a case in Chicago to finish when I got back from D.C. This was not a convenient time to feel anything less than 110%.

Besides, I had just completed my yearly physical. My doctor, who is also a lifelong friend, paraded me around his office telling everyone what great shape I was in. In fact, I was in good shape and had no idea of the news that was to come.

Forty-five days later, I started to get sores in my mouth. Bruises on my legs followed that I didn't understand. I lost ten pounds. I continued to feel tired. When I got back from Washington, I emailed John Capelli (my doctor) who became concerned immediately. He wanted me to come in right away.

Initially, I fought off the fatigue until I finished my Chicago case a week later. I can remember at times having trouble signing my name to the stipulations during the proceedings. A terrific young man, Steve Ziccarelli, had driven me back and forth to Chicago. He was concerned but I told him not to worry. I probably would feel like myself again once I got back to my normal workout routine.

After the Chicago case ended, I thought maybe I was just being a baby. That night I went out and ran three miles thinking the sores would go away. Maybe with a little discipline and hard work I'll feel fine and won't be as tired tomorrow? After all, I was 56 not 96 and took good care of myself. There was nothing hard work couldn't fix. Besides, I had no time to be sick.

The next day, my doctors' physician assistant called and wouldn't take "no" for an answer. John wants to see you. NOW! NOT after your next case! What could I really say? The previous night's jog had not miraculously cured me. I relented and drove to his office.

Admittedly, I was dizzy. My blood pressure was 60 over 40. The physician's assistant took it three times in disbelief. John took one look at my bruises and said I had leukemia. He wanted me to go straight to the hospital. I fought with him and told him I must have a spider bite that was screwing with my blood panels. To humor me, he drew blood and ran a quick lab at his office. My white blood count was ten times what is normal.

I agreed to go to the hospital after he called a mutual professional colleague for whom I had a lot of respect for as an oncologist. John put Dr. Malek Bandealy on speakerphone. He thought John was kidding at first when he heard I was the patient. He met us at the hospital later that afternoon.

My son Frank is my law partner. I had to call him to let him know I was going to the hospital for a test. The test was a bone marrow biopsy to determine the type of leukemia I had. We all met at the hospital. I was given the first of countless blood transfusions. I felt better and hoped all this cancer talk would just pass. The bone marrow biopsy revealed I had the worst kind of leukemia a 56-year-old man could have, Acute Myeloid Leukemia (AML).

The doctors asked if they could talk to my family. Frank was my health care power of attorney. I always wanted to be open and honest with everyone and felt my cancer diagnosis and treatment would be easier to handle if we were all on the same page. What I didn't know was what would come next.

The doctors told us that I probably had less than two months to live. They suggested that I start getting my affairs in order. Of course, there was always a chance for a cure but that was very unlikely. Later that night, I studied the literature and it said I had about a two percent chance of surviving.

I knew I was sick but really never thought I was going to die. The most upsetting news of the day may have been when the doctors said I would have to stay in the hospital for at least 30 days. For an active person like me, 30 days in the hospital sounded like a lifetime. In the end, my stay lasted 36.

Honestly, "Why Me?" did cross my mind. But there really wasn't any time for that kind of thinking. I had clients, bills and family to think about and I still didn't believe the doctors. I still didn't feel like I was dying.

THE NEWS

To tell my story, I have to introduce some of the main players. Many of you understand the emotions and consequences of being told your father, mother, brother, sister, significant other, spouse, or best friend has cancer. Unfortunately, some of you reading this book have had to break this news to your family members about your own condition. One of the toughest things about going through this experience is looking into the eyes of a grandson or granddaughter and thinking about all the mystery to unfold in their lives. I saw the look of fear on my children's, girlfriend's, and parents' faces. They had jumped on this voyage with me. My beating this cancer affected all their lives.

My parents **Frank and Carolyn Gagliardi** were in their mid-eighties when I was first diagnosed. They were in good health and felt very young when you consider their age. My parents were extremely involved in my life and the lives of my children and grandchildren. Of course, this was incredibly hard on them. Nana and Papa (as they're referred to in the family) have lived through a lot. Their families migrated from Italy without the comfort of money and basic things we take for granted. They came to a new country where the language and much of the culture was foreign to them. But their parents' challenges looked like nothing now compared to their own: the thought of losing their only child. It's every parent's worst nightmare.

Gennie is the oldest of my three children. She is a petite mixture of my mother and her mother, my ex-wife, Kathy. She has a degree in art and two sons, Vance and Stanley. She is an interesting concoction of fiery and stubborn Italian woman and peaceful artist rolled all into one. She is married to my son-in-law Kevin Gerou. Kevin is the co-author of this book as previously mentioned. Without his skill and creativity, my rambling thoughts would never have left my computer. Kevin is also a talented musician and writer. Coincidentally, Kevin was the school counselor at the high school located across from our law office at the time we worked on the book.

Frankie is named after my father. That is the Italian tradition. The first grandson is named after grandpa. Like I mentioned earlier, Frank is also my law partner. We have done a lot of things together. We hunted, fished, trained dogs, and did years of competitive baseball. He is married to my daughter-in-law Dana. Dana is a registered nurse. They have two beautiful daughters, Maya and Frankie.

My youngest son **Paulie** and I have also shared in a lot of these same hobbies. In fact, much of the time we all did these things together. Paulie was a very talented athlete who shares my same level of intensity when it comes to competition. He currently attends law school in San Diego where he lives with his fiancé Cristen and their dog Bocelli.

Nina was there for me when I needed her most. She was more than a girl friend to me. This was a relatively new relationship, although we had been friends for a long time before we dated. Nina is a very hard worker with three children of her own. She has a part-time job and operates a cleaning service. We'll talk relationships both family and otherwise in a chapter dedicated to relationships.

It's important to concentrate on those that you are the closest to first. It's best if you can tell them the news yourself although these are not easy conversations. It's easier if you think as I did, that you are not going to die. They all took it differently which I expected. Basically, I assured them I was going to be alright (but I knew it would take some time to convince them). After all, I was still getting used to the idea that something was wrong myself.

It didn't take long for others to find out. People were in shock. You've heard about things like bucket lists or the old question, "if you found out you were going to die, what would you do?" I tried to explain to everyone that I was a happy guy and had confidence that I would make it through this. Besides, I lived a busy - fun filled - challenging life.

Did I have some regrets? Sure, we all do but there wasn't time for that now and there really never was before. I tried to live under the adage of, "live every day like it was your last." I didn't put things off and fought for what I believed in. The mental attitude came easy for me. I want to win but am also sorry to admit... I think I just hate losing even more. Winning to me was making each day (no matter how many were left) a special one. I like that. I like fights I can't lose.

After my initial diagnosis, I was allowed to come home for a day or so before I started chemotherapy in Milwaukee. The first day I came home, Nina and my close friends Jeff and Betsy came over. They couldn't believe it. Betsy's sister had breast cancer and eventually passed on during my illness. I think this was exceptionally hard on her. It's hard on everyone that has had a loved one die from cancer. It brings back all the painful memories. You have to be aware that everyone will react differently. Each person's thought process is a result of his or her own past experiences.

Betsy cut my hair as my son Frank (who had stopped by), Jeff and Nina watched. Frank hadn't slept. His eyes were red and falling off his face. He wanted to move on things to make sure he did his lawyer part. He brought over a health care power of attorney and a statutory power of attorney to begin with. We all looked at each other. I said, "Frank, give me a chance, I am not going to die." I meant it. This helped settle everyone (I think). I wasn't ready to sell the farm. I assured all that if the time ever came, I would let them know. I wasn't trying to be stubborn.

I was lucky to have the love of the players in my life. Their love gave me strength. Kathy, my ex-wife and mother of our children, showed her concern as well. We had been married for over thirty years before our divorce. She was there for me now too. There are important things and there are more important things in life. A lesson I wanted to be able to continue to teach. I wanted everyone to have a common goal: treat each other with love. It doesn't always work but as you will read later: if we want our energy focused on getting well, we have to accept what comes our way and work on our health through positive thinking.

I know you probably have a list of people you would rather not see at this time. Remember, they need you as much as you need them. Let them in. I wanted my children to learn from my struggle and be prepared for their own life struggles. I felt stronger because I was teaching and overall, I considered that to be my life's work.

My experience could help enrich my life and help others understand that same message. Even though I never felt like I was dying, I did understand how sick I was. I understood how vulnerable I was to infection and even death. Although it's convenient at times, I don't believe in avoiding reality.

News traveled fast. I saw a lot of people in the couple of days before my treatment started. I felt strength and encouragement from their love and concern. I still kept thinking all I needed was a good night's sleep and I'd be OK again. Cancer was hard for me to accept. I wasn't used to being held back. It didn't help that I was a medical negligence trial lawyer. I know this can trouble some doctors but my team wasn't rattled by it. In fact, some were experts I used in my cases. They knew me as a fair and practical lawyer. I had a true concern for improving health care and lowering the cost of health care for everyone. At the time of my diagnosis, affordable health care was at the top of my list. People deserve this, not just the wealthy – everyone. I had just been to Capitol Hill screaming this mantra to every legislator that would talk to me as the state representative for the Wisconsin Association for Justice.

The responsibility of being President of the Wisconsin Trial Lawyers Association the next year was another thing that really concerned me. How could this happen right now? It is never a good time. Trust me on that. The longer we live, the more challenges we will face. This was just another one. Unfortunately, everyone was telling me it was my last one.

You can't get away from thinking about what will happen to the ones you love. It will be expensive. Ridiculously expensive and will there be anything left? Fortunately, I had given Kathy (my ex-wife) the debt free assets. Although we had our struggles and differences, it was very important to me that she was taken care of. Like any marriage, we had tough times but plenty of good ones too and had raised a family together.

Isn't that terrible to have to worry about money when your life is on the line? Although the financial complications of being sick couldn't be ignored, the money wasn't the big problem. I wanted to see my grandson Vance hit that home run. I wanted to see my granddaughter Maya sing a song at her first school recital. I simply still wanted to be here.

We were still struggling to get the law practice on its feet after several changes. My colleagues were great and helped us through a lot. Frank had to grow up as a lawyer quite fast. Frank had to face all this with the burden of everyone telling him that his dad was going to die. He wanted to sell everything. They must have taught him that in law school. I told him to let me go through this treatment and then we'll decide what to do. I am not going to die. Please believe me.

That's one of the toughest things. Once the news gets out, people don't know what to say. They don't have to say anything because you can see it on their faces. They had to wonder if it was the last time they would see me. Talk about awkward conversations, it's amazing. You still talk about sports. You still talk about the weather. Sometimes, it's just too hard or people just aren't comfortable facing the truth.

I didn't know that I was about to go to war with cancer. The tired feeling was from the leukemia beginning to simmer inside me. I thought maybe I just needed to cut out red meat and eat more fish. Our minds are interesting devices. We often believe what we want to. But if anything, I wanted to be the poster boy for good health care.

I wanted to be an example to everyone that we can fight cancer. Of course, I did not want to die. But if I did, I knew I had lived a good life and was grateful for all I had been given.

After all, Frank and Gennie had already given me two wonderful grandchildren in Vance and Maya (they would later give me two more, Frankie and Stanley). I had great kids and incredible parents. The most difficult thing about the news was the thought of putting all of them through this. You really don't have a choice though. Put your best shoes on and walk through this like any other struggle. The reality is you can become stronger by going through this process. I wanted to see my family grow and understand the simplicity of life.

Thank God for the players in my life. Just like in sports, a player has to have a good team to win it all. And I was confident that I had that. Even though I was a fairly stubborn and independent person, I knew that I couldn't get through this alone and that every person facing this battle should think about his or her own support system. Who might you need to reach out to in order to help fight this battle? Without the support of my family, friends, doctors, and girlfriend, I may not be writing this book right now.

NOT MY IDEA OF A VACATION!

When I started my long stay at the hospital, I tried to lighten people up the best I could. I never wore my hospital clothes and dressed up every day. I had them bring a desk into the hospital room so I could still work. It was important for me to keep my routine as regular as possible. No one found me lying in bed. I even had them bring me an exercise bike that I used a couple of times per day. Most of the time, I was either at my desk working, watching CNN from my chair, or on that exercise bike.

I kept track of my progress and amazingly, rarely even felt very sick. I actually got a lot done. I billed out my time to pay the bills and once everyone realized I wasn't about to give up, the news wasn't so bad. Heck, it wasn't so bad for me. I am being truthful. Nothing changed, just the color of the walls in my new office.

Later when I got out of the hospital, I even played golf with the I.V.P. tubes in my arms. One of the nurses told me to take the legging part of long socks and pull them over the I.V.P. tubes. This kept the I.V.P. tubes from rattling around when I did things. I played some of my best golf that way. My son Paulie has a YouTube movie of me. I bought a pair of nickers (ordered them when I was in the hospital over the internet) and got a" paper-boy" English themed hat to wear. I went to the golf course when I got out of jail (I mean the hospital) to play with the guys in my golf league dressed as an old time golfer. It lightened things up and was just some good fun.

It wasn't always as easy as I try to remember though. There were long hours spent alone in my room when the steroids kept me up most of the night. I wondered how long it would take to be back to my old self. I did get mad at times and hated wasting time. Although I tried to always see something good happening, it was a challenge to keep being productive. For those of you like me, who try to use every ounce of energy they have every day; chemotherapy puts a cramp in your style.

Also, people were dying all around me. I knew the nurses pretty well and even settled a case later on for one of my nurses I had during treatment. I was the constant source of legal information for the staff. The truth is: you can't imagine what good medicine it was for me to talk with them about their legal problems or questions. It helped fill the time and gave me a useful feeling. Like I mentioned, I can be a real pain in the ass when I am bored. Even though a lot of people wondered why I was so devoted to my work while facing a life and death situation, I had to be. Working was an important part of my treatment plan. It's important for patients to continue the things that make them feel happy and productive.

The news wasn't always pretty but you can't dwell on it. Once they give you the prognosis, what is there left to say? Really? Are you certain? Sure, the odds weren't good. In fact, the real odds were terrible. My advice is not to shy away from the truth though. The odds and percentages are true but they are just numbers. Who is to say what number you are? Someone has to be the two percent survivor. Why not you?

I have always liked craps. In craps, there are 36 combinations of two dice. There are six combinations of seven. This is compared to the number of combinations to roll the "point number" before you roll a seven. The point number is the number the shooter rolls on the "come out." The come out is the first roll of the shooter. If the shooter rolls a four, five, six, eight, nine or ten on the come out, that is the point. The shooter has to roll the point number again before he rolls a seven. If he makes his point number before he rolls a seven, he wins. This is called "a pass." If he rolls a seven before he makes his point number, he craps out (loses) and passes the dice to the next shooter. He keeps the dice until he craps out.

Casinos actually pay exact or real odds for the odds bet in craps. Every time a point is set, you can make an odds bet behind your original bet on the pass line. If four is the point, there are three chances to make a four compared to the six chances to make a seven. The odds are exactly two to one (which the casino pays if the shooter makes the point). I know this sounds confusing but it is a lot of fun once you do it a couple of times.

The point is: to go even up with a casino is really good. I like those odds. I also liked my odds at beating cancer. Remember that you can be your own handicapper when it comes to your chances. How you approach your illness and how positive you are affects the odds dramatically.

I am a firm believer that when we are born, we are also certain to die. We just don't know when.

PAUL GAGLIARDI

There is a timeline between birth and death and
we never get to know where we are on that timeline. It's a waste of your time and energy to be
afraid of dying. Once you die, your job is done.
You just die. It's that easy. Your work in this world
is done.

NANA'S SOUP

Everyone has a cure. I heard it all - from soup to nuts. It gets hard to listen to. You don't want to be rude but you know you need normal blood cells to live a healthy life.

My mother's (the Nana) soup is pretty famous. She makes chicken noodle with great big chunks of chicken and soft pasta shells in it. When facing a life and death situation, it's amazing how some of the little things in life can become so significant and others so trivial....that soup your mother is so proud to make for you and that you know was made with all her love....those goofy things the grandkids say that just bring a smile to your face and help you realize how simple and wonderful life can be. And you also realize how insignificant it is that someone cut you off in traffic that day or that someone didn't give you the best service when you were out to dinner.

For me, it was extremely important to understand what I was up against. That is just my personality. When I wanted to get better at golf, I read books, watched videos, video-recorded my swing and analyzed it. When I wanted to learn Italian, I put note cards all over my apartment labeling the Italian word for everything. You can call it a little crazy but that's my style. It's an important part of what makes me successful. I approached cancer the same way and wanted to be informed and discover anything that might help me overcome my illness.

Leukemia is the abnormal growth of the components of white blood cells. The white blood is made up of a number of components. A general rule is that they fight different types of infections. White blood cells are needed to fight all forms of infection, from bacteria to virus, to fungus.

The red blood carries other necessary goods we need to live. In particular the gases we breathe. Without a proper balance of red blood, we wouldn't get the oxygen we need to think, move, and exist.

Blast is an immature white blood cell. AML patients have excessive blast in their blood. Blood is formed in our bone marrow. If we just produce blast, there isn't room for the white blood cells that fight bacteria or the red blood cells, which among other things provide oxygen to our body.

AML doesn't sneak up on anyone. When it hits, it hits hard and fast. Within a relatively short time (weeks), it can become more than 85% of your blood volume. Normal amounts of blast are less than 10% of your blood volume.

When I initially went in to see my doctor, my blood pressure was 60 over 40. That is extremely low. I had been bleeding, bruising, was dizzy and fatigued. I also had a cold that wouldn't go away. All because I didn't have enough oxygen or platelets (red blood) or good white blood cells necessary to fight infections and viruses. The blast was in the 85% range. A bone marrow biopsy the next day confirmed the diagnosis.

The conventional and really only way to treat AML is to totally wipe out the bone marrow blood producing cells and hope that if you survive the chemotherapy, the blast is replaced by normal blood cells. Yes, the theory is pretty much that simple. It is similar in other types of cancer treatment too.

The chemotherapy kills the fastest growing cells. Blast is one of the fastest growing cells. We produce new blood cells all the time. Along with the blast, the chemotherapy stops hair from growing. Thus, the chemotherapy creates the bald look and your hair falls out. Nina and Gennie actually had fun pulling the clumps out.

The chemotherapy process (cycle) is repeated over and over (about once a month). The hope is that your body will return to producing normal cells and whatever caused it to get off the main road was destroyed.

Some of the success in surviving I believe is luck. The old saying is the harder I work, the luckier I get. There is some truth to that in fighting against cancer. Once you begin a cycle of chemotherapy, you wipe out your ability to fight infections and various viruses. Fungal infections can be even harder to over come.

After my third or fourth cycle, I got pneumonia. I didn't want to skip a cycle. Statistics had shown the number of cycles usually required for even a chance of being cured and I needed the next cycle to have a chance to be cured. This vacation was starting to look a little scary now.

It was a mess. I needed an endoscopy to biopsy some of my lung tissue to determine what type of pneumonia I had. If it was bacterial, I could take an antibiotic. There was enough time so that I could get strong enough for my next chemotherapy cycle. If it was a fungal or viral pneumonia, it could take a long time before I could begin chemotherapy again. Bacteria, fungus, and various viruses are everywhere. This is especially true in a hospital. You can wear a mask, but of course there is no guarantee that you will not catch anything.

In order to have an endoscopy you have to have sufficient platelets to survive the procedure. I unfortunately did not. Platelets are the portion of your red blood cells that allow your blood to thicken sufficiently to stop bleeding. This is why after a chemotherapy cycle, some patient's gums start to bleed for no apparent reason and won't stop. This happened to me on a number of occasions. This is dangerous because it means you need a blood transfusion immediately.

You have to have a sufficient platelet level to have an endoscopy. If it is absolutely necessary and your platelets are low, they try to pump healthy blood into you. Unfortunately, after a number of transfusions during chemotherapy, your body doesn't particularly want someone else's blood. That is where I was.

They attempted a transfusion of blood to bring up the platelet level and I had a bad reaction. My throat started to swell and I had hives. I started to choke. My parents were visiting and I didn't want to scare them. I reached over and closed the tube for the transfusion. I pressed the call button and waited for the nurse. The nurse was relieved that I had immediately stopped the transfusion. I was having an allergic reaction that could have closed my throat preventing me from breathing. The swelling and hives went away with time and Benadryl.

The doctors were waiting to do the endoscopy. The room was ready but I wasn't. I couldn't start my next chemotherapy cycle without treating the pneumonia. The Benadryl was started in a different IV. The Benadryl counteracts the allergic reaction. The lumps went down and breathing was easy again.

The IV Benadryl is the freakiest feeling of all the drugs. You drool, slur your words, and float into space. Cancer patients that need blood transfusions usually will experience oral Benadryl as a precaution. If they have a reaction, they will be given a much higher dose IV. My two cousins happened to walk into the hospital room right about the time they slowly injected the IV Benadryl. I know I freaked them out quite a bit. I tried to laugh it off and make them feel better but I knew that I sounded goofy. Later, my cousin told me they thought I was a goner.

I played golf with that same cousin the other day. I didn't shoot well but at least I played. You can't let the ups and downs get to you. Hang on. Fight the fight and use your energy wisely. You will need it. With the aid of Benadryl and some processed plasma, I was ready for the biopsy. The doctor was a saint. He waited around until they got my platelets high enough. It was a bacterium type pneumonia that fortunately responded quickly to antibiotics. I stayed pretty close to schedule with my cycles.

I was lucky. I thanked God and anyone else around for this good fortune. I wanted my chance to get in the ring with this cancer. I knew I had a couple of good punches left in me. One good right hand, I could put the cancer on its back for good. I needed that next chemotherapy cycle. Give me that chance. God did.

Nana's soup is important. The benefit isn't just for me. The soup makes Nana feel like she is doing all she can do. Patients forget that our illness affects everyone around us. They are helpless. Soups, vitamins and other remedy suggestions come in by the truckloads. As a patient, we understand the medicine because we have to. Without the soups and the love that go into them, we couldn't have the positive attitude we need to get well. Soups, attitude and blood transfusions are all medicines that become part of the cure. I loved them all with an open heart.

There is important nutrition in Nana's soup. Don't sell it short. Chemotherapy doesn't do a lot for your overall physical health. Nana's soup does. It gives you strength and that warmness we all need. Nana's soup can go a long way.

PAUL GAGLIARDI

WHEN YOU CAN'T MOVE

The first go around involves a pretty stiff cocktail of drugs when you begin chemotherapy for leukemia. They want to clean you out. You now enter the world of clean bone marrow. I have talked to a number of other cancer patients. Even though they have different types of treatment, they experience a lot of the same side effects.

About the third or fourth day, I awoke at 3am only to see my oncologist and several other white coats surrounding my bed. They all looked very concerned. I was a little confused because I felt fine. Actually, I was a little annoyed that they were screwing up my sleep.

I asked what brought them to my bedside. My doctor explained that I had a significant DIC issue going on. This is when your liver is over-loaded. It's an extremely serious condition. If the liver can't purify your body of poison, you can become toxic. In fact, you can become deathly toxic. My veterinarian friend Bill refers to this as "Death in Cage." Dogs normally don't survive this condition.

My oncologist was a little more optimistic. She said this was either really good news or really bad news. The good news could be that the chemotherapy was working and destroying all the cancer (bad) cells. My liver was over-working simply to rid my body of the cancer. The bad news could be that my liver couldn't handle the chemotherapy. That happens in older people. In cancer situations, if you are more than 55 years old, you are in the older category.

Since I didn't even feel weak, I couldn't understand what all the fuss was about. I told them that they should go home to their families. I would see them in the morning. I wanted to go to sleep but my assurances weren't enough for them. They stayed for hours until my liver levels started going down. This was the sure sign that my liver was ridding my body of cancer cells. As time went on, there was less and less to process. Then they went home. They were dedicated, good doctors. All is well I thought and went back to sleep for a couple of hours.

It wasn't always like that. I mean there were times I couldn't move a finger. I remember the experience of having a bone marrow biopsy after my first chemotherapy cycle was completed. I have a bulging disk in by lower back. During this vulnerable time, the area where they harvested the bone marrow from became inflamed and irritated the pre-existing bulging disk. The doctor who had treated me for my back was also at St. Luke's. He had seen me in the lounge area when I first started treatment. He was shocked to see me in the hospital. He said if I needed anything to let him know. I laughed and told him that I felt great.

Shortly thereafter, my back began to spasm. My legs started to shake. They rolled me in for an MRI and called the back surgeon. He did something to settle the inflammation and my legs calmed down along with myself. But for a time, I couldn't move. I guess I did need him.

I didn't know it then, but this was to happen more often than I care to remember. There were times when I would spike a fever for no reason. Neutropenic fevers are common after chemotherapy. You are immune compromised. With no defense system, your body's normal bacteria can set off an internal infection causing your body temperature to go up.

I remember lying in bed with the television on trying to go to sleep and feeling feverish. The nurses check you all the time and I did in fact have a fever. They eventually call in the infectious disease team and start you on IV's. On a couple occasions, I can remember wanting to change the channel on the television remote and nothing moved. It sounds crazy but sometimes you are that incredibly weak. I tried to explain it to Gennie. She probably thought I was crazy. I stopped trying to explain it after that. Everything seemed to have drained out of me. I didn't even feel like talking. I'm not even sure I even could have.

I continued to have some problems like that even when I was finally able to go home. I had developed a colon infection called diverticulitis. I was so weak I couldn't move. You lie there and wonder what's next. I was too stubborn to live with anyone or have anyone stay with me. Nina would try to help but she had children that she was caring for. Gennie wanted to be there but she had children too. My mother and father wanted me to stay with them, but I couldn't impose on them. They would have loved to but it wouldn't be fair. I felt bad enough getting sick and making them worry already.

PAUL GAGLIARDI

My mother and Gennie do yoga. I had spent some time doing yoga as well. I love physical and mental fitness. The paralyzed sensation felt like being in a total meditation state. Actually, I kind of liked it. Now that I am well, I can't repeat it! I have tried to reach what I would call a total state of relaxation but it just doesn't happen. At times, I thought: is this it? Is this the end? I remember thinking that if it was, it actually feels pretty good.

IT CAN HAPPEN

I am talking about death, dying, and the last good-bye. Whenever someone mentions the cancer word, the first thing people think about is death. He or she is going to die. OMG.

It can happen and many of us have watched a close friend or family member die from cancer. If you are a cancer victim (and more and more of us are if we live long enough), it is even more profound. How do I deal with this?

I watched family members and friends die from cancer. I was there at the end. I watched life leave them. I saw into their eyes just before they took their last breath. I saw wives and children say good-bye one last time. "I love you." "You are not alone." But you know deep down, they are alone because they make that trip without you. You wonder how you would feel. How will you act? What will it be like?

Of course, I didn't know what dying would feel like. And I tried to not even think that way because I knew it wouldn't help me beat cancer. I felt great when I touched the people I loved. I felt warm and good. Food was still nourishing. I wanted to go to work. I wanted the Brewers and Packers to win. Even faced with death, I would still get upset when they lost!

The long and short of it was: I was still myself. How could I be dying if I was still being me? I saw people in the hospital die during my stay. You would hear someone say that the family had said good-bye and he or she died peacefully.

He or she fought a good fight. What a shame to die so young.

It really wasn't until a couple years later that it hit me. After my struggles with post-chemotherapy, I realized how much I missed the body I once had. When I visited a family member about to enter Hospice, it wasn't easy to watch her struggle to breathe. She couldn't even swallow by reflex. The morphine had stripped her of her awareness. Her skin was cold and damp. I saw how I was supposed to die. She was a strong woman. She was a much better person than me. Why did death take away her dignity? Why is death so difficult?

My father who is the source of a lot of my logic and strength always told me that when it is your time, it is your time. He saw death at its cruelest moments. He was a medic during World War II. He did things that no human should ever have to do. He treated soldiers that were blown up in the fields. Often, more than half of the bodies of these soldiers were burnt. He told me, that the deadly smell of their burnt skin has never left him. I help veterans whenever I can. Even today, my son Frank and I helped two World War II veteran brothers. The one brother was never the same after the war. He was in the major battles in the South Pacific. He suffered from Post Traumatic Stress Disorder. Survivors' guilt is tough. I think I have a little of this.

Why do I digress about death in a book that is supposed to provide insight into beating cancer? Obviously, no one beats the inevitable. Everyone eventually dies. Death is part of life. What is important is how you live your life with cancer. You do the best you can with what you have. I can tell you what my uncle told me, "Winners never quit and quitters never win." This is true. Living a life that doesn't deny the truth is a key to surviving. My uncle died of cancer. We were close. I had a painting done of a small boy climbing a wall with those words written on it. His picture and mine were on the painting. When I gave this to him during his fight with cancer, I had no idea how much it would mean to me today.

We all die. The problem with cancer is that it makes the process quicker. Live each day to the best of your ability. Set reasonable goals. Make sure you don't have to be superman to reach your goals. I try to tell myself each morning that I am going to be the best person I can be today. Even when I make one mistake after the next, I accept it and know that it will happen. Maybe that was the best I could be that day. No matter what, I know the sun comes up tomorrow and I get another chance. I have control of my own attitude and appreciation for what is given to me. I'm the one who will decide what kind of day that I'm going to have.

You have control of your ability to smile. If you can help someone else smile, why not. You've done a good thing. I tried to make my family smile as much as I could when battling cancer. They think because you have cancer, you should be sad. Guess what? They are dying too. We all are. We just don't know when.

OTHER SCARY STUFF

Don't kid yourself. There are other scary moments too. The first bone marrow biopsy is scary because you don't know what to expect but it really isn't that bad. I even had one without anesthesia. That definitely hurt a little but it didn't last long and you can get up and just go to work afterward. Nonetheless, I would recommend the anesthesia. Why put yourself through it if you don't have to?

The direct line in your arm is scary. I didn't like the idea of someone putting a tube in my vein all the way to my heart and being awake to watch. What if they went too far? These nurses who are trained to do this are special. They know what they are doing and really don't hurt you. I had it done three times. It wasn't that bad.

Every blood test you have is scary. The anxiety of waiting for the results is tough. Is it back? Am I getting better? Is there an end to this? Not easy stuff to think about. For me, this was the worse.

It is really hard to deal with watching the friends you make in therapy relapse and die. Some people really felt they were next and unfortunately a lot of them were. For me, I felt guilty. Why was I doing well and they weren't? It didn't seem fair.

A scary part for me was the finances. I was at a low point when I was diagnosed and cancer certainly didn't make it any easier. I worked as much as I could. I would go to the clinic for chemotherapy early in the morning and stay until lunch. I didn't have an appetite but forced myself to eat because I needed strength to go to the office. Then, I would return to the hospital at night for a second dose of chemotherapy. That would go on for a week at a time. I tried to work during the therapy but I had to have staff read over what I did. I was afraid that I could have made some mistakes.

It was scary to forget things. My mind wasn't as sharp as it had been. It is coming back now but the process has been tough. Even though I am grateful that my mind is coming back, it isn't a pleasant thought to realize you were only operating on a half tank during treatment and for some time after. Don't be frustrated, that only makes it worse. Be grateful that you can think at all and work at ways to double check what you are doing. The double-checking process fortifies the thinking process and helps you think more clearly. Attitude is a word that is emphasized in athletics. It is especially important to cancer patients as well.

It was scary to wonder if I would regain all of my strength and stamina. What did I lose? Mentally? Physically? Part of your life is given up even if you survive. How hard should I push myself? All questions, even today, I ask myself often. Is the glass half empty or full? I am glad I have a glass. It doesn't really matter if it is half empty or half full. As long as you have a glass, you are still in the game.

The more you understand about your illness, the better off you are. Don't be afraid to ask questions. Don't be afraid to read everything you can. Talk to people. I felt the more transparent I was, the better it was for me and for those I loved. That is how I approached this. Some people are the opposite and I respect that. It is important to be yourself.

You are still who you are even with cancer. Once you accept that, you aren't as scared. Cancer should not have made me someone else. I just want to be myself. I wanted to do the same things I always did. Try to stay as normal as you can. It is best not to feel sorry for yourself. You are moving forward. You do change, as do the things around you. That isn't just because of cancer. Life changes and cancer is just part of the changes. You can't fight the current or you won't have enough energy to get well. Get to tomorrow and fight some more. Try to use the current to get you where you need to be. Healthy and strong!

WHO AM I?

Sounds like a silly question, but it isn't. You drop 20% of your weight in a couple of weeks. The hair falling out in clumps is even faster. So you just shave the leftover patches off. I can only imagine how that must be for women. In my case, a lot of guys my age are bald or shave their heads to be in style. No big deal.

Nonetheless, these changes in appearance are noticeable. However, that is the small change you have to face. The mental and physical changes are much more significant. Getting up in the morning is like the morning after polishing off most of that bottle of scotch your cousin gave you for Christmas. Remember how that feels? You had to struggle to remember what you were celebrating the night before. Worse yet, who was I with? What did I say? Whom did I say it to? Oh my God, did I make a fool out of myself? These experiences hopefully are few and far in between.

Unfortunately, alcohol and chemotherapy have a lot in common. They are poison. After a bad hang over, you can swear to yourself, it will never happen again. You do not have that choice with chemotherapy. As a matter of fact, you often have to go back for more the same day after struggling to get out of bed and trying to remember what yesterday was about. That is an uninvited change that you are told simply to accept. Don't expect anyone to understand. They won't. It isn't their job to understand. It is your job to get through.

They asked if I drank before the chemotherapy started. I said socially (even though I hate that response). I think drinking is more anti-social than social. I have seen, as we all have, drinking ruin people's lives. Regardless, the doctors told me that because I drank alcohol and didn't have bad reactions to it, my liver was somewhat preconditioned for chemotherapy. They were right. I didn't get sick from alcohol. I rarely had hangovers from alcohol. I handled chemotherapy in a similar fashion. No vomiting. I had occasional bowel issues that mushroomed into a portion of my bowel being infected. The infected portion was eventually removed through surgery. Fortunately, I tolerated the chemotherapy remarkably well. Some of us weren't so lucky. You must stay focused and understand that you will get through regardless of how bad the food tastes.

What people didn't see (or at least were kind enough not to say anything about) was the weakness in my legs, the lower back and arm pain; the numbness down my leg, the forgetfulness, the vision problems and the sleepless nights. It changes you a lot. I just never wanted to admit it. I went to work and pushed to be better than ever. I just thought there weren't a lot of options. I looked at it as another challenge. After all, this would end one way or the other. They said I had thirty to sixty days left. There was no time to complain.

The truth is: I didn't know where I was going. At times, I didn't recognize myself. The people who love you are kind. They allow you to pretend everything is fine. If you keep smiling while you pray, it is a lot easier. I can assure you of that. Prayers can keep you focused on the hope for a better life. Prayers are uplifting and remind us of how lucky we are to be given a chance to spiritually improve ourselves regardless of what is happening within our bodies. By improving spiritually you give yourself worth and are continuing to live. This is strong medicine.

I didn't give the down side of things very much thought. Negative thinking just got in the way of getting things done. I have always been an end-result guy. The process is to get to the end. Stuff like pain or weakness just got in the way to getting done with the treatment. I didn't have any time for this. If I got a fever, they put me in the hospital. They made me stay until whatever infection I had disappeared. I knew the fever could be the end of me. A recent friend who was turning the corner on leukemia went into the hospital with a fever. We thought she would be out in a day. She was a lot younger than me. Normally, at her age, she would have the strength to survive and fight another day. She had the same great doctors I had. It was difficult for me to attend the funeral service.

I always thought the body heals over time no matter what I do. If enough time went by, I would be better. I did smart things. I ate healthy. I tried to get enough rest to let my body heal whether it was a cold or knee surgery. If I needed to be medicated, I did what the doctors said.

Chemotherapy doesn't work that way. It is a constant pounding to kill off all of the fast-growing cells in your body. Stomp out the fast-growing cancer cells to the point they give up. The collateral damage is part of the war. You have to be up and standing for each new battle. There are casualties. I lost some of my hearing. My vision from the steroids is worse. I have glaucoma. Steroids send the eye pressure up especially for glaucoma patients. This kills part of the optic nerve. You lose peripheral vision. I only have 60% of my optic nerve left. This is a hassle and no one wants to drive with me. I see things in time but a fraction later than everyone else. Everyone jumps and covers up thinking I didn't see the car coming. I see the car. This isn't easy for my passengers to understand.

I have appreciated everyone's patience though. Some of the changes are embarrassing. I am sure this is also the process of aging. We all have to adjust but the question is when. A gradual adjustment would be nice. Cancer patients do not have control over the amount of adjustments they need to make after chemotherapy. There is no time to complain. Make the adjustments.

Most important, you feel tired and frustrated. The old cure was one good night's sleep. That doesn't cut it after chemotherapy. You can sleep all day and night and still feel like someone threw a wet blanket over you. I just tried to push harder and get used to it. I tried different foods, vitamins, and changes in exercise. I set goals. First, I'll try to walk six blocks. Then, I moved up to a mile. Then walk a mile and jog for

ten minutes and so on. The goals help take away
the pain of knowing a lot has been taken from you.
Focus on one goal at a time. This helps a lot. I
knew making it too tomorrow was important.
Something I should be satisfied with but I just
wanted more and still do.

It isn't easy. There is no exact lesson plan.
There are setbacks you don't anticipate. I recently
had to have a steroid injection in my back. I had an
inflammation and couldn't walk. The pain was
severe in my right leg. I had this in smaller doses
than my first round in the hospital. This time I
knew I needed some help. I probably pushed too
hard on the treadmill. Where is the happy
medium? This was just another setback to learn
from.

If you have someone you can talk to, that
may also be very helpful. I didn't have that kind of
time. I wanted to move forward. I did do a lot of
reading. I tried to write down what I was feeling.
That helped too. I hoped letting others know what
I made it through might help them in their time of
need. It was therapeutic for me. The good Lord
helps those that help themselves. I like to add, not
only help themselves, but others along the way.

It all happens so fast you don't notice all the
changes that the outside world is seeing. This is
especially true if you are busy trying to get back to
the old you. I really didn't realize how weak I was
until I started getting stronger again. I don't
believe you are ever "the old you". Times changed.
You changed. My goal was to be a better version
of the old me. If I could not be who I was, I should

at least try to be someone better than the old me. That gave me hope.

Make it as much fun as you can. I didn't have the strength to physically do a lot of things I used to do. In my pre-cancer days, I often didn't find the time to enjoy reading. I didn't always go out to dinner and entertainment afterwards. So, when things slowed for me, I did a lot of the things I had missed out on. I started reading more. I wanted to play my guitar again. I began working on my electric train set for the grandkids. Doing these things made a difference to me. I felt lucky to find the energy to do them.

I didn't sit and feel sorry for myself because everyone else could do things I enjoyed that I couldn't do anymore. There was a lot I could do and I tried to be happy with that. Life is defined by the choices we make. That doesn't change simply because we have cancer.

Personally, I think strength comes from within. I wanted everyone to feel strong with me. I wanted them to know I was doing fine and I would be there for them if they needed me. My doctors told me that stress is self-inflicted. Stress distracts the body's healing power. It strips you of strength. You need everything you have to withstand the treatment. Finding ways to live and work around the treatment is important to maintaining the mindset for a happy and productive day. I think that goes a long way to finding yourself while going through treatment.

Maybe no one knows who he or she is because we change every day. It is how we change that makes us who we are each day. Cancer is a challenge as is chemotherapy. It is a change. It changes you. You can't be afraid to go with some of the flow. Sometimes you can use the current instead of fighting it. When you are down, every bit of energy helps. Don't fight yourself. Be proud of everything that is a part of you. Keep trying to change for the better. It gives you a purpose.

PAUL GAGLIARDI

ALL THAT GLITTERS IS NOT GOLD

This chapter is a little flash forward. I was reading some of the chronicles that I put together during my illness. It has now been almost two and a half years since my post-induction therapy bone marrow biopsy was normal. As a rule of thumb, after two years of remission, AML doesn't relapse. In layperson's terms, you are cured. They still watch over you. I see my oncologist every two months right now. My last blood tests showed almost normal white blood counts. The lack of normal blood levels isn't from the cancer; it is from the chemotherapy. At almost sixty years old, my oncologist was very pleased to see my blood levels continue to move into the normal ranges.

No one is quite sure why I keep getting better and stronger. I can only explain what I am doing. There are definitely ups and downs of my routine. I'll try to explain...

The mornings are still very difficult. I do not bounce out of bed excited to be alive and wanting to go to work. I get up. Take a couple of Excedrin. Turn the television on. Eat a bowl of cereal. Watch a little more television (usually flipping between Mike and Mike [ESPN] and the Good Morning America show).

After my shower, I am pretty much awake. I have one cup of coffee in the morning when I get to the office and usually read the paper. I really don't kick into gear until about 8:30am or 9:00am even though I have been up for a couple of hours.

Presently, I go to a chiropractor two times a week for strength and balance. I think I am making good progress. Depending on my work schedule, I have lunch with my friend Bill. Then I go back to work. I work until 5:00pm or later and then try to hit some golf balls or practice putting. In the winter, it is just back to work.

After getting home, I try to do the treadmill or elliptical every day for about 35 minutes with some free weights mixed in. I settle down to do my reading and emails. Then go to bed around 11:00pm. The workouts need to be tempered due to a bad back and achy bones.

That may sound like a regular day. But before I got sick, I got up almost two hours earlier and went to bed an hour later. Granted, this may be a part of old age sneaking in. Because of the timing though, I think it has something to do with the chemotherapy. As my blood keeps getting closer to normal (especially the hemoglobin) I have more energy and strength. I keep hoping it continues to inch forward. It takes three steps forward and two steps back. That still keeps me going forward and provides some hope.

I was a lot worse before I had bowel resection surgery four months ago. I kept getting a bowel infection about once a month. I think it never really went away after the first infection. It just simmered inside me. Chemotherapy had created a vulnerable spot in my bowel. It made me irregular. Something I hated. I could not go to court without worrying that I would have to run to the men's room.

After about four hospitalizations, I begged the surgical team to take out the bad part that we believe was irritated by the auto compromise effect of chemotherapy. They would not do surgery at first because they worried about my prognosis. I was supposed to be dead. Why would they do surgery?

My oncologist stood up for me, as did my general doctor. Finally, we did this and I have been getting stronger all the time. I am actually at my normal weight again. As a former wrestler in high school and college, that means a lot to me. I have good strong moments again. It is like the country song that refers to the cowboy who can't do all the things he once could but he is still the same man for one time. It is funny how you relate to certain songs.

Here's the thing. After chemotherapy, depending on your age, you recover. You get your hair back. You can see your body returning to form. You gain your weight back. Your color improves. Your stamina starts to return. It is never fast enough so you have to be patient and set reasonable goals. You have to realize there will be setbacks. Not many things in life go up in a straight line. Every chart or graph has its bumps and regressions along the way.

Little things get in the way. It seems like every little ache or pain is doubled. I started doing bench press (even though I have a bad shoulder). Once it gets irritated, it takes forever to settle down. I modify my routine to compensate. I want my strength back. Not to fight someone in a dark alley but to feel good. To hit a golf ball the way I once could. I want that part of me as long as I can have it. I am willing to work hard and sacrifice to get there.

My back flares up because I try to run on the treadmill too hard. The next day, my legs ached and my back at times was so sore I could not get comfortably into my car. I try not to tell anyone. They would think I was crazy to try to run on the treadmill or outdoors. How do you explain that something precious has been stolen from you and you want it back? I compromised. Now I walk the first ten minutes. I move up the speed ever so slowly, then cool down and walk some more.

The elliptical is only so good for you after chemotherapy. Yes, it gets your cardio up for the 35 minutes or so you do it. It is a fixed exercise. No wobbling. When you walk or work, you wobble. Those muscles are weak from chemotherapy. You need balance. My chiropractor has plates that vibrate when you walk on them. This helps with balance. It also loosens some of the stiffness and helps with the soreness. He also has a couple of strength machines that you just push on and the computer measures how you are doing.

Like I mentioned previously, seeing for me is one of the real challenges. I had inherited glaucoma. The glaucoma was kept under control with eye drops. The medicine kept the eye pressures within reasonable limits. Once the pressure is high, it puts too much stress on the optic nerve. The nerve or part of it dies leaving your eyesight limited to right down the middle. It becomes more and more narrow. When you are on chemotherapy, you have to take steroids.

Steroids increase the optic pressure. I didn't realize this until I had an eye exam after I had been in remission for a while and was done with chemotherapy. My pressures were in the mid-thirties. That is high. We got it down to the mid-teens with additional medication. But some damage was done. I lost 40% of my optic nerve.

Driving is harder. I can't see what is next to me. I have to move my head to see what is along side of me. It drives people nuts when they ride with me. My buddy, Bill, who is a veterinarian, explained to me that dogs just adjust to this. That's what I am doing. It is working but I also need the right lens to assist in seeing better. For someone who hates to waste time, it is frustrating. It's the little things.

I keep reminding myself nothing is straight up or down. The chiropractor monitors the progress. I see some but it is slow. Patience has never been my strong suit. I know I have to take little steps if I want to win this battle. Every time I try to take the big steps and run out of the blocks, I am backed up a number of weeks. Trust me, one day at a time and one step at a time. That is easier said than done.

That is the physical side. The mental side is not much better. You get tired faster. No one performs well when they're tired. I was a multi-task type person. I did not feel right if I was not using every moment to its fullest. Chemotherapy makes multi-tasking harder. You do not know where you left your pen. What did I want to say? Gone. I keep losing my blue tooth. It is embarrassing. My letters are not to the point some times. Communication skills are not as sharp.

I play mind games. If I cannot remember something like a name of a person, I go through the alphabet. A - Albert, Alfred; B - Ben, Bill; C - Chuck, Casey. D - Dave. Yeah that's it. David Jones. Bingo. Believe it or not, that is getting better.

Reading is tough. At first I could not read interrogatory responses for any length of time. I had someone look over everything I did. I am much better. I keep at it. I want to get stronger mentally. I tell myself to take it one day at a time. I have to remind myself of where I was and the improvements I've made when I get frustrated.

I can't give you any words of wisdom. You get a chance to live. I say make the most of it. It is not easy. For me, I had little choice. A number of people depended on me. I had to get back in the game and fast. Even if you are financially set, you still want to be the person you were. There is no easy way out. If you were one tough "hombre" before chemotherapy, you need to channel that toughness. You need to be tougher inside more than ever. You need to be determined. Most important, you need patience to think clearly and gain back your physical strength.

Do not forget that we are not getting younger. Eat the best foods you can. Exercise routinely. Keep your mind on a program to multitask again.

These are not secrets. No one wants to be here if given a choice. One day at a time - one foot in front of the other. The result, we hope for - one smile after the next.

Sorry, the grandkids are coming to trick or treat and I have to do the elliptical today and shower before they get here. We all have priorities. If grandkids knew what they do for a sick ole man, they would bottle it and sell it to pay for college. Stop reading and go for a long walk. Better yet, give someone you love a hug. Enjoy.

RELATIONSHIPS

I find this to be the most interesting but possibly the toughest of all areas living with and surviving cancer. In life, everything we do revolves around relationships. Relationships contain all the elements of life. Hope, love, pain and anxiety; they're all there. We've already covered how important it is to avoid stress when you are fighting cancer. Stress saps your strength more than anything else. Stress is harder on you than chemotherapy. So when fighting cancer you don't need to be in relationship battles that can drain needed strength and focus.

Relationships can vary depending on if it's family, a friend, or your significant other. Each relationship has its own dynamics. You want your family and friends to understand that you need to focus your energy on the battle. You hope they accept and follow this but they too can only do the best that they can. They often have a lot on their plate in addition to your illness. Their life is continuing just like yours is.

Most important, relationships grow and change with time. At least the good ones do. I am referring to the ones that are worth your energy. Relationships help you to grow as a person. If we can keep growing as a person while we are fighting cancer, we are still living. We are still accomplishing something important. It helps give value to your life with cancer. It adds worth during a very difficult and challenging time for the patient and the people who love you.

Relationships revolve around a number of things. Cancer can be a stumbling block or it can open a door that was previously shut. I learned a lot about myself through the relationships with those I love. And not everything was rosy. If you are lucky enough to survive, I hope that some of the insight that follows helps you have a better life after struggling with cancer. Remember, as a cancer patient, you aren't the only victim. There are people who suffer your pain and anxiety with you through it all.

We show our best and worse side to those we are closest to. This is especially true when we are vulnerable. Cancer brings its share of stress to everyone. Everyone is vulnerable during this time. Some of the closest people in your life will treat you the same before, during and after your illness. This could be good or bad. You hope all will forgive whatever you have done to hurt them before cancer but it doesn't always happen that way.

For those of you that want to hold a grudge, whether you are the patient or the family of the patient, please reconsider. You only have so much time in life to be together. I would hope if nothing else, one of the benefits we can receive by way of this health struggle is the life lesson to love and let those we love be themselves. To truly live, we must learn to forgive. Forgiveness opens the heart for healing. It allows family to focus on healing. Do not waste energy on issues that are in the past. There is no benefit to going over the past. It only gets in the way of healing. Cancer is a tough opponent that does not need any help. If you are the cancer patient, learning to forgive even in a day-to-day situation is of utmost importance to your survival.

I recently heard the inspirational late coach Jimmy Valvano's speech that he gave during the kickoff ceremony to his V Foundation. As many times that I have heard the speech before, it never gets old for me. He was a special man. He lived life with enthusiasm. I was a big North Carolina State fan when he coached there. He fought cancer the same way that he coached; with enthusiasm. He always wanted to make a difference in the lives of those he loved and every person he met.

If you keep holding on to a grudge, it's ultimately you who loses. You are cheating yourself and losing a chance to make up and enjoy what remains of your life. Jimmy was a big time winner. His life was cut short by most people's standards. Not by mine though because he lived large. He gave it his all - all the time. One day in his way of life may be more than eighty years for those that don't understand how to love and forgive.

Some people will be there for you after your diagnosis. You think whatever the wall was between you and them is no longer there. You feel their love and sincerity. Some do see the light because the thought of losing a loved one matures them. They realize how vulnerable life is.

If you do recover though, some people will still harbor deep negative feelings that resurface. This is hard to believe, but true. You must continue to shine the light of love and forgiveness. You hope they eventually will see it. It is never too late and one day of love is better than a lifetime of hate. There are some that want to forgive everything once they know your days are numbered and many people will return to the way they felt about you before you were sick.

None of this means they don't love you. They all do. It is just part of life. Try to kindle the warm feelings. Especially during cancer and chemotherapy, we need to use the love from relationships into strength. We also have to let go of the stress that trying to constantly fix relationships brings. We need to concentrate on fixing our health, plain and simple. Hopefully, those that love us realize this. We, the patient, need to set this example for everyone to follow though.

I spent a lot of time thinking about how to make things better for those close to me. Should I keep things from them so they wouldn't worry? Should I select what to tell them and try to control the information flow to make it easier? You are able to do a lot of thinking while on chemotherapy because the steroids keep you up hours on end. It seems like your mind never stops.

Rule #1: Don't try to control the outflow of information. Tell the truth to those in your inner-circle and let them have access to all the information. To do otherwise makes an unfair situation even worse. Plus, who can keep up with all that? Your job is to fight for your life. You can't waste vital energy figuring out what they can handle and what they can't. If you die, they have to handle that. Let them in and be fair. I signed health care power of attorney forms so that everyone could ask any question or look at any record they wanted to. I sent group emails to my parents, children and Nina letting them know what updates I received from doctors as soon as possible to avoid anxiety. I believe this was helpful and they confirmed to me that it indeed was.

I always expected to live into my mid-nineties like my grandfathers did. Drink wine and take Metamucil. My grandfathers' theory to longevity was a shot of whisky in the morning, Metamucil before bed, and another shot to sleep well. Instructions I received independently from both of them when I turned sixteen. I followed the Metamucil and shot before I went to bed advice. The shot in the morning was not for me. Hey, they told me if you want to learn how to bake bread go to a baker. If you want to learn how to live long, just ask an old man like they were. It made sense to me. We never had to talk about cancer though. Now I was on my own.

Many of those close to me didn't change their attitude when I was sick. It hasn't changed now either. This was really amazing. Count your blessings for those around you who are strong. Be grateful. From that gratitude comes strength. You will need to put the pieces of your life back together hopefully if you survive. These same family members and friends will be there for you. You can rely on their consistency. This group loves you and would do anything for you before, during and after cancer. Nothing changed.

Each person has a different dynamic. And anyone that has had or been around children knows that they are all different. I felt my children's pain. I had always been there for them and their mother. This was new territory but I was determined not to make them stop their lives for my illness. If I died, I'd be gone. Thank God for life insurance. Have a nice life without me. Of course, that isn't what they wanted. I was "Grampee". Or just "Pees" as my grandsons often referred to me as.

What is important is your faith in what you did before you had cancer. If you brought your kids up doing what you thought was best, then you have to have faith that they will do what is best for them and their family. That is as good as it gets. You certainly can't control the situation other than being as strong as you can. Don't try to control them. You barely have enough energy to try to control what you have to do to fight. Your children love you and don't want to lose you. They will be there in their own way. Just be loving and forgiving. It is hard to do sometimes, but this is the only way. That doesn't mean you stop being a parent. You say what needs to be said with the internal caveat that we trust them to do what is right for them. We only say what we say because that is a parent's job.

I have great children. They are very different. I love all of them the same. I try to spend my time with all of them as well as the grandchildren. I could not be more proud of them. My philosophy with my children was similar to how I interacted with the doctors. For the most part, I told them every day I felt good. In my mind, I actually did feel pretty good. I told them that I am going to be better than ever.

One of my greatest pleasures is seeing how
my children are good partners to their significant
others. They all get it. They will have good families
and lives because of it and that is the most
important thing. I think this is one of the things
that helped me accept my fate. I felt my children
were really good people. They also had chosen
good life partners. Who could ask for anything
more even I lived another fifty years? This gave me
a lot of strength.

To have someone to survive for makes a big
difference. To want to do well financially,
physically, and mentally gives you the drive to
fight. Thinking about a comfortable life with Nina
and having the desire to help everyone in the
family gave me strength. No small task but it was a
goal I had set. Having that goal helped me get up
in the morning when I thought I couldn't.

You have to have goals. There is nothing
more powerful than your love for a partner (soul
mate) to help give you the strength and energy to
fight for your life. For that, I will always be thankful
to Nina. If you are in a good relationship, whether
you are married or simply friends, relationships
give strength and meaning to life. We need to
cultivate our relationships especially when life is
threatened as it is in cancer.

Men don't understand women. Women
sometimes do not understand men. There have
been songs, movies and poems about a man's love
for his partner. When a man loves a woman, she is
the most beautiful thing on earth. She doesn't
need make up. There is no such thing as ten extra
pounds. She will always be in the eyes of her soul

mate, the beautiful woman he fell in love with. She doesn't age. She only gets more beautiful. I am not sure women understand this. A man in love would do anything to have his woman see herself through his eyes. If she could, she would be the most confident person on earth.

Women see their children this way. This only happens a few times for a man, if at all, in a lifetime. I see it in my sons. That gives me great joy. I had it for Kathy and Nina. I know how lucky I am to have felt this way. The beauty of the people you love can also fill you with strength. There is no way to explain this. It is simply good medicine.

Let me know if it works for you. I feel like I am starting over. My law practice, my kids and grand kids, all are new and challenging. In my personal life, I am trying every day to be a better person. I sometimes think, my God, did I fight so hard for this? Did I fight so hard to start everything over? You fight hard for the chance to ask yourself those questions. One day at a time. Actually, starting over and trying to be a better person is a good reason to live.

Remember, no one will really know what you went through. It doesn't matter. It is history. Today is a new day. Move on. Try to do the best you can just like you did every day you were in treatment. Do not expect too much. Make your expectations realistic. Good luck my friend.

PAUL GAGLIARDI

FAITH

There are no two people who have the identical faith. Faith is an extremely personal feeling. I grew up Catholic and went to private schools all the way through high school. Later, I graduated from a Jesuit College and Law School. I was an altar boy, took religion in school, and took religious philosophy courses in college. I read the Bible - both Testaments. I was part of prayer groups and used to pray before my wrestling matches or just through some of the tough challenges that life brings. But none of this prepared me for the challenge of facing death.

I had a very humble feeling. Nothing I was going to do could stop this cancer if the doctors were right. If I turned to God now, would he laugh at me? Now you want my help? When it was easy for you, where was I in your life?

I don't think that is how a supreme being thinks though. That is how we think because we are imperfect. We are not all forgiving. We are not capable of understanding the wealth of knowledge it takes to be fair and loving. After all, we are just people or servants. For once, I was glad to be helpless. I was glad to have my fate in the hands of someone supreme to me. I didn't have to think this through. It was just the way it was. It was comforting in many ways.

I felt it wasn't right during this time of need to look to God. I felt He had more important things to attend to. I was a speck in the universe. But, I prayed. First, I would say the Hail Mary. Then, I'd concentrate on the Lord's Prayer... forgiving those that "trespassed against me." The Act of Contrition may have been the most important knowing I had sinned and asking for forgiveness. God never came and spoke to me. He was there. He allowed me to believe I could fight and win. I didn't need to re-read the Book of Job or anything like that. I didn't think God was punishing me. I was thankful for what he gave me in life. He gave me patience to fight and the strength to continue to help others. That is my calling and gift.

My friend Bill is probably one of the best friends a person could have. A few years back his wife died of cancer. Kathy was a wonderful woman. She was a special kind of wife. Bill loved her and appreciated her. Shortly after Kathy's death, our mutual friend Jerry died of cancer. Bill brought him to Mayo for a checkup after Bill was concerned something was wrong. This was especially hard on Bill's son Ben. Jerry was Ben's godfather. Ben referred to Jerry and me as Uncle Jerry and Uncle Paul.

Within months of Jerry's death, I was diagnosed and received a death sentence. Once again, Bill was there for me as he had been for Kathy and Jerry. Fortunately, Bill had also met a wonderful woman named Sarah after his wife's death and she was there for me as well.

Bill is Lutheran. He gave me a Lutheran Bible to read. I found out it is much like the Catholic Bible. Not much was different except for the person reading it. Me. My son Paulie had also started attending a Bible group. We had many interesting discussions on faith that I appreciated very much.

PAUL GAGLIARDI

Bill reminded me that there is nothing wrong with turning to faith in the time of need. We all do. It is natural. I needed someone to say that when Bill did. I think he knew that. I was truly amazed at the number of people who said they were praying for me. The electricity of prayer can light a country. In my case, it lit up my heart. Their prayers helped give me the strength I needed to fight my illness.

Never underestimate the power of prayer. It is the most positive emotion of all. It gives hope. Hope is a virtue right next to love and charity. That comfort relieves stress and allows you to fight the cancer instead of the natural fear of losing the battle. Your faith gives you strength.

Everyone has his or her own way. I respect all beliefs. I respect the right not to believe in a supreme power. For those that don't believe, I am here to tell you, I felt the love in all the prayers for me. That was real. It was very strong medicine.

I will never be able to repay those that prayed for me and helped save my life. It is the most humbling experience. I only hope I can give something back to those that gave me so much. My college roommate, Tony and I have always remained close. He is in New Jersey and of course I am in Wisconsin. He lived in Wisconsin with me for a while when he worked for a company here. He has always been in medical sales.

Tony belongs to the Knights of Columbus. He goes to church every Sunday. Tony talks to his God. His life-style and religion is his. If it works for Tony, no pun intended, God Bless him. He has had his share of struggles.

Tony, like Bill, has never pushed his religion or beliefs on me. Tony has pushed other thoughts and opinions. He isn't short on that, but not religion. We talk every day and try to support one another. We had our reunion for Boston College after I was diagnosed and taking chemotherapy. He put our friends on the phone all night just to say hello to me and wish me well. I couldn't make the reunion, but from my chair, I was sort of there. It is these things that help get you through. You feel like your life really didn't stop even if it did.

I have another friend who belongs to AA. The twelve steps are important to him. He doesn't preach them. If you weren't close to him, you wouldn't know he was a recovering alcoholic. I have met others who are very pushy with their beliefs. We all know them. They feel it is their duty in life to convert the world. I believe, if it works for you, you are lucky and should stay with it.

This Christmas, my mother gave me the Book of Job to read. I have mixed feelings about the book and the time it was written in. The main message to never give up and that misfortune doesn't mean that God is punishing you is true. I think the Supreme Power has much more important things to consider than my health.

Blaming anything or anybody for your cancer is a mistake. Again, this takes away from the energy necessary to focus on getting well. I hate to say tunnel vision is what you need but it is. This is from a guy that has been a multi-task guy all of his life. I don't want to miss anything. But this one time,

your energy needs to be spent on getting well. No
time for blame. Job was right. God doesn't punish.
He loves us all. Love is stronger than any form of
blame or hate. Have patience and let your positive
thinking help heal your body. Thus, the "Patience
of Job."

DON'T BEAT YOURSELF

There is a lot to be said about common sense. We often put common sense on the shelf when we need it most. Why we discount this valuable commodity in the time of need is something I can't explain. There are a number of challenges when fighting cancer. A little dose of common sense can go a long way in this fight.

My friend Bill attributes my analytical thought process to being an accountant in my first professional life. Balancing all those debits against the credits. I like to think of it as common sense. Balancing the potential benefit against the overall risk when making decisions.

To understand my approach to fighting cancer, you have to start with the brain that we are all born with. Science tells us that the brain takes up 2% of the body's mass. Not much you say? I agree until you go a little further. The brain cells use 20% of the oxygen we breathe and burns 25% of the glucose we digest. I admit, this makes the brain a greedy little organ. If you are like me, you want a bang for your buck. So I say, use the gray mass. God must have placed considerable importance on the brain to provide so much of our lifeline stables, oxygen and sugar, for brain consumption.

First act of common sense tells me not to argue with our Creator. My feeling is, He knows what He is doing. The next step is to put it to best use.

PAUL GAGLIARDI

I recently read a book by a former memory champion from the United States. Basically, the competition consists of memorizing a deck of cards in less than two minutes; faces and names, poems, and strings of numbers. Each of these tasks alone are pretty amazing. The author, Josha Foer, was a young journalist who decided after covering the event for a publication, he would give it a try. He had several good coaches and worked very hard to achieve this remarkable accomplishment.

` Josha's approach was scientific with the right mixture of common sense. The real message is that we all have the talent to improve our brains including our memory. We have to treat our brain the same way an athlete trains for a sporting event. In fact, the memory participants are referred to as mental athletes.

Many things happen to you when you are told the reality of cancer. In my case, the odds were not very good for a permanent remission. This news clouds your thinking, as it is extremely hard not to think about. In my case, I applied common sense. Common sense told me that I didn't feel like I was dying. I surely didn't want to be preoccupied with dying. Whatever time was left, I wanted to live doing what I enjoyed and what would be worth remembering. I looked at dying in the same fashion I always did. I know death and taxes were sure to happen. We know when April 15 rolls around. We don't have the benefit of knowing when our last day will be. Regardless, if cancer was going to take days from me, I wasn't going to help cancer ruin whatever days were left.

I made up my mind to continue to live my life as full of love and happiness as I could.

We also know that chemotherapy is brutal on all of our organs, not just our brains. However, the term we often hear is "Chemo Brain". What is chemo brain? Chemo brain in part is the fog we are in because we are thinking this is the last time I will see my grandson. I wonder what he will grow up to be? This is consuming our thoughts. Who cares where the keys are or if I turned the stove off. That's part of it. The other part is we are not getting the oxygen and glucose to our brain that our brain needs to perform at 100% because of what we are going through.

Common sense told me to exercise to increase my heart rate forcing my blood to provide greater quantities of oxygen throughout my body. Common sense told me to eat the right foods that didn't become instant fat. Glucose not immediately used for energy is stored as fat. The right balance of sugar helps keep the blood glucose at its most efficient level. That means less work for the rest of the organs. This is a critical time. Most cancer patients lose large amounts of body mass. The body is using up the fat for the necessary additional energy to fight cancer. By eating smart, your body will have an easier time rounding up the energy to fight cancer. Additionally, your brain isn't taking a beating always fighting for more oxygen and glucose. You have more energy and can do more of the things that you always did. Thus, you have naturally offset some of the depressing aspects of cancer. My favorite common sense rule, win - win. When the decision results in a win - win situation, it is a no brainer (no pun intended).

Once you reach remission, you must battle the plateau wall. The same rules apply. You think this is it. I will never be able to run again. I will never be able to work like I used to. Nonsense! When a runner hits a plateau, she/he breaks down his training. More sprint work. Different diet. Change my sleep habits. Smaller parts result in bigger results. Fighting cancer or cancer recovery plateaus is the same challenge.

Most of us trying to get our health back are older. We don't want to work out after or before work. It is hard enough to go to work and then contribute to a family at home. Common sense allows us to break down our time and prioritize what we need to do. What will help us the most. The better shape we are in, the more energy we have for work. The more energy we have for work the better off we should be financially if we are using our time and energy wisely. Some things are out of our control.

Patience is the other factor that we have to learn and master. Something I have great pains trying to integrate into my lifestyle. The better off we are financially the less stress we have at home with our family. Things do not always fall into place before, during and after your battle with cancer. We can't blame ours or the person we love's health for everything that happens. It is part of this thing called life. We have to patiently walk through these ups and downs.

Life also will always have plateaus. We never will have a free pass to the end line. It will always be a challenge. We have to find a way to enjoy the challenge. Make the fight into memorable moments that will represent our lives.

I have a number of Korean friends. My friend John is a Karate instructor. The memory I have when John had the unenviable task of trying to train me was, "Little step by little step." The actual translation was, "Steppie by Steppie." You have to imagine John saying this with his Korean accent for the full affect. To this day, I hear John saying this when I rush through something without any patience. My inner voice says, "OK John, 'Stepie by Steppie,' I get it."

In summary, that means taking care of your body and mind. Feed the greedy beast between your ears and make it work for you. Exercise common sense. Stay focused on the end line to have a better life.

LOOKING BACK

First and foremost, to have an opportunity to look back is very special. I know I am lucky. I want to make the most of this good fortune.

Is there a reason for my survival? Some of my doctors told me I had been preparing all my life for this challenge. I did the things people should do for good health.

I don't think it was just the physical preparation that mattered. All of my life, I tried to maximize each moment of life. I wanted to be happy. I wanted to share my happiness. I wanted to always be hopeful. I wanted to show people that in their time of need, there is light at the end of the tunnel. It doesn't always work that way. We all have dark moments. I tried to keep this attitude when I was told I had cancer. It helped me feel alive. I would suggest that attitude before, during and after cancer. It is a better way to enjoy the life we are given. It is part of the medicine that prepares us for challenges. Cancer is just another challenge.

Some of my clients suggested that I am alive to serve them. I survived to win their cases and be their advocate. Could it be that genetically, I am simply within the 2% that survives at my age?

I think it was all of the above. The secret ingredient is to use your time efficiently. You need to focus on getting well. Don't do things that work against you. Do the things that provide you with energy: eat a healthy diet of lean protein meats, fruits, and vegetables, sleep enough, and avoid stress as much as possible.

Most important, think positively. I believed I was going to beat my cancer. If not, I was willing to make the best of every minute I had left. No one was going to cheat me and especially not myself.

A car can still hit me. I can get a different type of cancer. We never know where we are at on the timeline of life. How far away is death? Your guess is as good as mine.

The effects of chemotherapy and every day challenges don't just go away. That isn't how life works. There are always challenges. There are always obstacles. Just because you had cancer or are still fighting cancer doesn't mean the everyday challenges disappear. They are there. Hopefully your fight against cancer has made you a tougher warrior and lesser challenges are easy to face now.

Right when I thought everything was in the past, I recently (more than two years past my last chemotherapy treatment) hit another bump. I had worked 80 hours the week before. Wow, the old me. I made some money for the people I love. Wow, the old me. I felt great. My mind was multi-tasking. I could read through statutes and case law with intelligence and speed again. Wow, the old me.

Not so fast. I got out of bed and I fell on my face. My right leg felt numb. Then the radiating pain set in. I couldn't walk. The timing is never good. I still had a lot of shopping to do for the holidays. I had an episode in the hospital where after the first round of chemotherapy they did a bone marrow biopsy. After the biopsy, my leg started to shake. The pain was severe. The MRI revealed three levels of dried out inter-space discs. I also had a bad disk that was irritated by the biopsy. They told me that can happen. But they treated me successfully. Frankly, with all that went on, I really didn't think much about it.

Later, as I started to try to work out and regain strength, I would get some neuropathy down the same leg. I experienced numbness and pain down my leg from time to time. My doctor had me go to the chiropractor. This is a young former baseball player that my son Frank played baseball with. He is great. He started me on traction once a week. It seemed to work.

Thinking I was doing fine, I stopped the traction. We shifted our attention toward his Strength 4 Life program. This is a computer-designed program that is quite safe. Not much movement and monitored resistance to develop strength in the chest, arms and legs. I, in turn, at home turned up the treadmill and the elliptical. All the pounding and stopping the traction caused the neuropathy to return ten times more. I didn't realize the effect this would have on the herniated disk in my back. In part, this was from age and in part, from chemotherapy. I didn't realize that I was overdoing it. It is time to turn in the Nike shoes and buy a stationary bike. No more pressure on the spine.

My prayer is that I can avoid the spinal fusion surgery. My advice is to think through everything. Listen to your body. I was about to start P 90X. In my mind, I wasn't getting in shape fast enough. I wanted to make up for the two and one-half years of life I was robbed of.

Be real and face the truth. Some is my age. Some is chemotherapy. But most important, listen to your body and take care of it. After all, you don't have to be a genius to know you were given another chance. Be grateful and not foolish.

The best advice anyone can give to cancer patients (and their loved ones) is to love each other every day. Be as strong as you can. Consider yourself lucky for finding this love for each other. Not everyone does. If you find it, cancer or not, you are one of the lucky ones.

Don't forget your dreams when you were in a dark place. I wanted to see the grandkids grow and become adults. That was my dream. If you are alive you are living the dream. How good is that?

I hope this book some how makes your trip through cancer and chemotherapy easier. That was my intention. My best to you and maybe someday we will meet. P

PAUL GAGLIARDI

ABOUT THE AUTHOR

Paul Gagliardi is a lawyer whose office is located in Paddock Lake, Wisconsin. He lives nearby in a country setting close to where he raised his children. He is the father of three and the grandfather of four so far.

He continues to do his life work as a trial lawyer. Whenever he can, he strives to encourage those facing challenges such as cancer. He believes helping others gives him the strength to live every day to its fullest.

www.ingramcontent.com/pod-product-compliance
Lightning Source LLC
Chambersburg PA
CBHW060205290526
45789CB00003B/1172